# BLOOD PRESSURE:
Questions You Have ... Answers You Need

## Other titles in this series:

ARTHRITIS: *Questions You Have ... Answers You Need*
ASTHMA: *Questions You Have ... Answers You Need*
DEPRESSION: *Questions You Have ... Answers You Need*
DIABETES: *Questions You Have ... Answers You Need*
HEARING LOSS: *Questions You Have ... Answers You Need*
PROSTATE: *Questions You Have ... Answers You Need*
VITAMINS AND MINERALS: *Questions You Have ... Answers You Need*
HEART DISEASE: *Questions You Have ... Answers You Need*

## By the same author:

HEART DISEASE: *Questions You Have ... Answers You Need*

# BLOOD PRESSURE:

Questions You Have ... Answers You Need

## Karla Morales

*Consultant editor Dr Robert Youngson*

**Thorsons**
*An Imprint of HarperCollinsPublishers*

Thorsons
An Imprint of HarperCollins*Publishers*
77–85 Fulham Palace Road,
Hammersmith, London W6 8JB
1160 Battery Street,
San Francisco, California 94111-1213

Published by Thorsons 1997
3 5 7 9 10 8 6 4 2

© The People's Medical Society 1984, 1991, 1992, 1997

The People's Medical Society asserts the moral right to
be identified as the author of this work

A catalogue record for this book
is available from the British Library

ISBN 0 7225 3314 4

Printed and bound in Great Britain by
Caledonian Book Manufacturing Ltd, Glasgow

All rights reserved. No part of this publication may be
reproduced, stored in a retrieval system, or transmitted,
in any form or by any means, electronic, mechanical,
photocopying, recording or otherwise, without the prior
permission of the publishers.

# CONTENTS

| | |
|---|---|
| Publisher's Note | vii |
| Introduction | ix |
| Questions and Answers | 1 |
| Information and Mutual Aid Groups | 56 |
| Glossary | 57 |
| Selected Bibliography | 66 |
| Index | 69 |

# PUBLISHER'S NOTE

No popular medical book, however detailed, can ever be considered a substitute for consultation with, or the advice of, a qualified doctor. You will find much in this book that may be of the greatest importance to your health and wellbeing, but the book is not intended to replace your doctor or to discourage you from seeking his or her advice.

If anything in this book leads you to suppose that you may be suffering from the conditions with which it is concerned, you are urged to see your doctor without delay.

Every effort has been made to ensure that the contents of this book reflect current medical opinion and that it is as up to date as possible, but it does not claim to contain the last word on any medical matter.

Terms printed in **boldface** can be found in the Glossary, beginning on *page 57*. Only the first mention of the word in the text is emboldened.

# INTRODUCTION

Few of us give much thought to the condition of our arteries until we learn, often by bitter experience, just how important this is. Yet one very common arterial disease – atherosclerosis – is, in our pampered western society, by far the most common cause of death and severe disability. Atherosclerosis has, with very good reason, been called 'the number one killer of the western world'. It kills far more people than cancer does, and it kills and maims by narrowing arteries so that the heart, brain, other internal organs and limbs are deprived of the blood that carries to them vital oxygen and nutrients. The result is heart attacks (coronary thromboses), strokes, organ malfunction and gangrene of the extremities.

Atherosclerosis cannot be diagnosed without special imaging tests such as contrast angiography, but the disease is closely associated with one change in the body that can easily and cheaply be measured – blood pressure.

Abnormally high blood pressure is one of the

principal risk factors for heart attacks and strokes. This is no coincidence: High blood pressure damages the linings of the arteries and predisposes a person to developing atherosclerosis. In turn, and especially in older people, atherosclerosis can cause high blood pressure.

For these reasons you need be in no doubt about the importance of the subject of this book. High blood pressure is a killer, and you owe it to yourself to know as much about it as you can. This is even more so as the condition gives no hint of its presence until it is at a dangerously advanced stage. Reading this book could save your life.

Dr R. M. Youngson, Series Editor<br>
London, 1997

# QUESTIONS AND ANSWERS

**Q** **What exactly *is* blood pressure?**
**A**  It's the force your heart exerts on the blood in your arteries to drive it round your circulatory system. When your heart beats – when that portion of your heart called the **left ventricle** contracts – oxygenated blood is literally shot into your arteries.

In its travels through your body, your blood presses against the walls of the blood vessels it is passing through. The vessels stretch and contract to maintain blood flow. If the vessels are narrowed or rigid, increasing the resistance to blood flow, blood pressure rises.

When it comes to measuring blood pressure and expressing it in numbers everybody can understand, there are two sets of readings. When the left ventricle contracts and the blood's force against the vessel walls is at its greatest strength, you have what is called **systolic** pressure. After that contraction, when the heart is more or less in its resting phase, the blood pressure is lower. This resting or relaxation pressure – the pressure in the

# BLOOD PRESSURE

arteries just before the next heartbeat – is known as the **diastolic** pressure.

Blood pressure readings, then, come in two numbers. For example, 120/80 (expressed as '120 over 80'), 150/95, and so on. The first number is the systolic, the second number is the diastolic. The difference between the two readings is known as the **pulse pressure.**

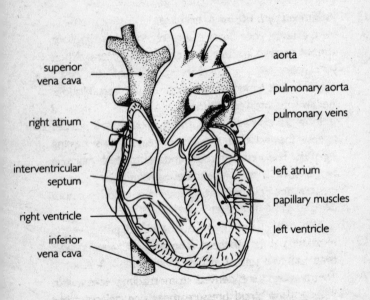

# QUESTIONS AND ANSWERS

**Q** **Which of the blood pressure numbers is more important – the systolic or the diastolic?**

**A** Both are of interest and concern to doctors, but the one they seem most interested and concerned about – the one that starts the bells ringing and the lights flashing – has, traditionally, been the diastolic.

**Q** **What is normal blood pressure?**

**A** 'Normal' is always a relative term when it comes to the way human beings function. Taking body function measurements isn't like taking a history examination: There aren't any 'correct' answers and no 'perfect' scores. A lot depends on a whole host of conditions.

According to prevailing wisdom, a reading of about 120 systolic over 60–90 diastolic is 'normal'. But you'd be hard pressed to find anybody with exactly 120/80 pressure, or with exactly 120/80 all the time. The 120/80 measurement is an average of quite a wide range of readings. Various times of the day, activities or emotional states can raise or lower the reading without being a sign that anything is wrong.

**Q** **How do you get these numbers – 120 over 80, and such – anyway?**

**A** The numbers are derived from readings taken with the standard blood pressure measuring device, called a **sphygmomanometer** (pronounced *sfig-mo-mah-nom-i-tur* – an awkward mouthful, isn't it?). If you've ever had a physical examination, you've met up with a

# BLOOD PRESSURE

sphygmomanometer. Most people refer to it simply as a **blood pressure machine**.

The way it works is this: A wide band, or cuff, is wrapped round your upper arm. The cuff is then inflated by air pressure. The same air pressure pushes a column of liquid mercury (*Hg* is the scientist's abbreviation for mercury) up along a numbered scale that is measured in millimetres (usually abbreviated as *mm*).

A stethoscope is placed against your arm's artery, known as the **brachial artery**. When the cuff has been inflated enough to cut off circulation to the lower part of this brachial artery, the person listening through the stethoscope (which is placed against the artery at the crook of the arm) will hear no sound. As the pressure is slowly released, the cuff loosens, the blood begins to flow again into the lower artery, and the column of mercury falls. The pressure in the cuff is now just a little below the peak pressure in the artery. At the point when the stethoscope can pick up the tapping of the heartbeat in the artery, the millimetre level of mercury indicates a figure approximately equal to the systolic pressure. Soon, as the pressure in the cuff is further released, the beating sound gets louder, then either fades gradually or ceases suddenly. The number on the millimetre scale at that point is approximately that of the diastolic pressure.

So if your blood pressure is 120/80, or 120 mm Hg/80 mm Hg, what that means is that your systolic pressure was detected, pinpointed and measured when the column of mercury was at a height of 120 millimetres, and your diastolic pressure was detected, pinpointed and measured when the column of mercury was at a height of 80 millimetres. These numbers merely represent a convenient method of noting and comparing blood pressures.

**Q Are blood pressure readings with a sphygmomanometer accurate?**

A They're close, but not perfect. While other more accurate measurement methods exist, they are far too complicated and invasive for general use in the doctor's surgery. For the most part, a sphygmomanometer reading is actually somewhat lower than the true arterial pressure.

Another problem with this indirect method of determining blood pressure is that you can get incorrect readings if you don't carry out the procedure exactly right. For example, if you don't pump the cuff tight enough – and, thus, don't entirely flatten and close off the brachial artery – you'll get a reading that's too low. The same goes if you let the air out too quickly, or if you use an adult-size cuff on children or adults with very thin arms. You might get a false high reading if a person's arm is too thick for the standard cuff. That's why some obese people who don't have high blood pressure seem to – it's not their blood pressure, it's the inadequate size of the cuff that's providing the false reading. The width of the cuff must be greater than two-thirds of the diameter of the arm, and the length of the bit that inflates should be more than two-thirds of the circumference of the arm.

Should you try to take your own reading at home, it could be way off if you take your pressure with your arm resting on a table or in some other elevated position – the cuff ought to be at heart level, and the best way to do that is if the arm is kept down at your side.

In today's booming self-care market, most new, low-cost blood pressure measuring devices are not the mercury column type of sphygmomanometer. Instead they have gauges or digital readouts. While the mercury column types are still considered the best, most accurate and most durable, they are a bit more complicated to use without help and they are more expensive. The new digital readout electronic pressure gauges can do well enough if they are, first, well-made, and second, taken care of – and, perhaps, occasionally serviced, if possible.

Don't forget to ask your health practitioner if his or her sphygmomanometer has been checked for accuracy and serviced lately. Incidents of surgery sphygmomanometers being way off – and thus affecting treatment options – are more common than you might think.

Q  **When is a blood pressure reading considered high blood pressure?**

A  Again, it's a fuzzy area. According to the medical experts, when blood pressure remains at or over 140/90 over a period of time (usually at least two readings over three days, or after several hours' rest) in people under 40 years of age, that's **high blood**

**pressure**, or **hypertension**. In people over 40, 160/95 puts you into the danger zone. The reason you need to have your blood pressure measured several times over a few days – or even a couple of times in one visit – is that nervousness, real or imagined intimidation by doctor or staff, stress or other factors can raise your blood pressure momentarily. To accept a single reading as significant would not take into account blood pressure's normal, everyday ups and downs.

**Labile hypertension** is the name given to this fluctuating kind of high blood pressure. People whose blood pressure is easily affected by the stress of a medical examination are, of course, more likely than average to experience blood pressure rises from the ordinary stresses of living. Doctors, however, do not agree on the question of labile hypertension. Some say there is no such thing. **Sustained hypertension** means you have it all the time. Labile can become sustained if not taken care of.

**Q** **Is high blood pressure a disease?**
**A** Definitely.

**Q** **What causes it?**
**A** Here's an answer you're going to hear a lot during the course of this book: Nobody knows for sure. It may be due to one thing or it may have 'multifactorial aetiology' – doctors' jargon for lots of different causes and reasons. Heredity is one factor, although that only explains transmission, not cause. Diseases of the kidney

are prime culprits. The brain chemical acetylcholine has been linked to hypertension, as has something called the natriuretic hormone. **Sleep apnoea** – a sudden stoppage of breathing during the night – may cause high blood pressure in older men (although it might be the other way round; nobody knows for sure). Environmental conditions have also been implicated. It could be all or one or none – always, sometimes, or never. That's what makes high blood pressure so hard to fight and to make generalities about – and to write routine prescriptions for.

Q   **Is high blood pressure a common disease?**
A   It certainly is. Around 15 million people in Britain and 61 million in the US have it. But only about half of those know they have it.

Q   **How can people not know they have high blood pressure? What are the symptoms?**
A   That's the point – for the great majority of people with high blood pressure there are no symptoms at all. And when those few that do exist turn up, it's usually only after the blood pressure is very high already. That's why they call it the silent killer. The only way to know if you have high blood pressure is to have your pressure checked.

High blood pressure is implicated in many of the deaths and disabilities resulting from **strokes**. Thirty-seven per cent of men and 51 per cent of women who die of heart disease are known to have had recorded blood pressure of over 140/90 on at least three occasions. In Britain, every year about 100,000 people have a first stroke, and strokes cause the death of about one person in 100 at the age of 40, and one person in 10 at the age of 75. Nearly all the strokes in the elderly are related to high blood pressure. About 80 per cent of strokes are due to obstruction of a brain artery, 10 per cent to bleeding within the brain, and 10 per cent to bleeding around the brain (sub-arachnoid haemorrhage). **Heart attacks** and strokes together cause twice as many deaths as cancer.

Q **You mean there are absolutely no symptoms?**
A Well ... there are very few absolutes these days. What might be possible symptoms of high blood pressure vary from person to person, and they could be symptoms of other health problems as well. But ... severe high blood pressure is too dangerous to take any risks, and most doctors say that if you're having headaches, heart palpitations, a flushed face, blurry vision, nosebleeds, a hard time catching your breath after exertion, fatigue, **tinnitus** (a ringing or buzzing in the ears), **vertigo** (the feeling that you or the world is spinning dizzily), or any combination of these – well, then have your blood pressure checked to see if that's the problem.

Q **Can high blood pressure be cured?**
A Well, yes and no. **Primary** or **essential hypertension** (85 to 95 per cent of all cases) is the kind of high blood pressure that seems to happen either because of

heredity or other unknown or hard-to-find factors. This kind of hypertension doesn't have a cure, but it is controllable through various means and procedures that we'll talk about soon. Essential hypertension is a by-product of one or several malfunctions in the body's system of checks and balances which regulates pressure in the arteries.

**Secondary hypertension** occurs as an offshoot of some other condition, very often kidney disease. (The kidneys, in terms of high blood pressure, can be either culprits or victims; that is, either the kidney problems can cause high blood pressure or high blood pressure can cause kidney problems. Either way, the renal [kidney] system is among the first to be considered when hypertension is present.) By controlling or curing the basic problem, secondary hypertension may just disappear.

Q **What can happen if my high blood pressure goes undetected and untreated?**

A Besides the aforementioned stroke, high blood pressure is a pathway leading to heart attack, **congestive heart failure**, or **coronary artery disease**, and other high speed exit ramps from this life. By making the heart work harder to push blood through the arteries, high blood pressure – in the form of **hypertensive heart disease** – can make the heart grow in size and at the same time tire it out, with unhappy consequences. Further, it's believed that the increase in blood pressure eases the way for fatty deposits to build up on the artery walls and eventually clog them.

Reducing hypertension pays big dividends. A recent study of 37,000 people reported in the British medical journal *Lancet* found that for every 5 to 6 millimetres of mercury by which a person's blood pressure is reduced, the risk of heart disease declines by 20 to 25 per cent and the risk of stroke by 30 to 40 per cent.

**Q** **If my GP tells me my high blood pressure is 'benign' or 'mild', does that mean I have nothing to worry about?**

**A** **Benign hypertension** means that your hypertension isn't **accelerated** or **malignant**, two extremely serious stages of the disease. However, as pointed out in the textbook *Principles of Internal Medicine*, 'hypertension is never truly benign, since even mild elevations of diastolic pressure are associated with increased risks of premature death and of vascular complications involving eyes, brain, heart, and kidneys.'

**Q** **Are men more likely than women to have high blood pressure? Black people more than white?**

**A** According to most research, hypertension occurs almost twice as frequently in black people as in whites, and black people suffer more illness and death from their elevated blood pressure. High blood pressure can be found more often in white men under 50 than white women of the same age, but after 50 it's just the reverse. Among black people there is no difference in occurrence between men and women. About a quarter of all white people over 65 have high blood pressure; this percentage is 50 per cent for black people.

**Q  Is blood pressure affected by the weather? By the changing seasons?**

A  There is some evidence that it might be so for certain people. If you have normal blood pressure, there's no seasonal variation. However, according to researchers at the Department of Medicine and Geriatrics of Osaka University Medical School in Japan, people with essential hypertension can expect slightly higher blood pressure in winter than in summer. The reason given for this is complicated and mere educated guessing.

**Q  During a physical examination, my doctor looked in my eyes to see if I had high blood pressure. Why?**

A  High blood pressure causes changes in the **retina** – from constriction of the tiny arteries (arterioles) to a condition involving bleeding and optic damage. The retina is the only place in the human body where the arterioles can be looked at directly. As a result of a retinal examination, a medical practitioner can gain a lot of information about which stage of hypertension a person is in and what needs to be done. The worse the changes in the retina, the worse the outlook.

**Q  Does blood pressure go up when you get older?**

A  It doesn't have to, but it often does. And when it does, it's frequently related to 'hardening of the arteries' – which affects the elasticity of the arteries, the flow of blood through them, and the increased pressure on the more rigid vessel walls. **Atherosclerosis** – the most common cause of hardening of the arteries and the major cause of stroke and heart attack in Britain and the US – are trademarks of high blood pressure and a major cause of ill health. This is because not only does high blood pressure lead to the development and worsening of atherosclerosis, but the worsening of this dangerous disease can then lead to higher blood pressure readings. Blood pressure going up with age might also be related to the weight we put on as we get older.

While a certain changeability in systolic pressure is to be expected – in extreme cases, systolic pressure shoots up past 200 mm Hg in about one tenth of all older people – diastolic pressure should not change with age.

**Q Can nervousness raise my blood pressure?**
**A** It can, especially if it's a long-term nervousness, or what is normally called chronic anxiety.

It is entirely normal for any worrying situation to cause the blood pressure to rise. Such anxiety causes the heart to beat more rapidly and more strongly.

But whether the raised blood pressure associated with anxiety is likely to cause permanent hypertension is quite another matter. Chronic anxiety is not generally cited as a significant cause of hypertension. At the same time, most doctors would acknowledge that persistently raised blood pressure can, at least in theory, damage the arteries in a manner liable to lead to hypertension. It may surprise you to learn that many doctors do not accept the widespread view that stress causes permanently high blood pressure. This idea is frequently expressed in popular medical literature, but you will not find it in medical textbooks. Of course, stressful events will certainly raise the blood pressure temporarily.

Q **Isn't stress primarily a problem of the workplace?**

A Not at all. Home pressures, family problems, money problems, even excessive noise are all stressful situations which can lead to temporary high blood pressure. Even game-playing stresses can do it – blood pressure can rise like a guided missile while a person is playing a video game. In a person with existing hypertension, such rises can be dangerous. At least one video game-related high blood pressure death is on record.

Q **If stress is potentially dangerous, what can I do to de-stress myself?**

A If you do have raised blood pressure, your doctor might put you on antihypertensive medication and let it go at that, or perhaps urge you to exercise to work off your nervous energy.

On the other hand, certain kinds of behavioural therapies have been shown to work. Deep-breathing relaxation training, in combination with diet and sodium (salt) reduction, has allowed many people to go off their medication completely with no risk. **Biofeedback** is another technique of tuning in to the body's own calming rhythms that has met with success, as has progressive muscular relaxation.

Meditation is a well-known relaxer, and studies performed and reported by researchers employed by the transcendental meditation movement claim that the systolic blood pressure of people who meditate are significantly lower than the blood pressure of same-age non-meditators.

Studies also show conclusively that owning a pet, or merely watching fish swim in a tank, can do wonders for your blood pressure health.

Behavioural therapists certainly can be recommended by your doctor. The other forms of relaxation may not exactly be your GP's cup of tea. You can probably get a lead on these techniques, and others, by consulting the Yellow Pages.

The Chinese knew about behavioural therapy for high blood pressure long before it had a fancy medical name like hypertension. Ancient Chinese doctors recommended 'placidity under all circumstances'. It's a theory that may work as well today as it did back then.

**Q Can people with high blood pressure exercise safely?**
A Not only can most high blood pressure sufferers exercise safely, but the exercise can bring their blood pressure down. You just shouldn't overdo it. Hypertensives not on medication can exercise moderately – walking, jogging or swimming – with safety and to their advantage. The exercise ought to have weight loss as its goal.

It's hard to say for certain if exercise alone lowers blood pressure. The drop could be the result of exercise-induced weight loss or a change in body sodium levels. But that's for scientists to argue over. If it does some good, it's worth doing, even without knowing all the whys and wherefores.

**Aerobic exercise** can benefit cases of mild and moderate high blood pressure, but doubts have been expressed about the safety of **isometric exercise**. The pushing, grunting and straining of the isometric resistance routines have been viewed traditionally as blood pressure elevators. However, more recent studies have suggested that these dangers may have been exaggerated. If you are hypertensive it would be wise to discuss this with your doctor before getting into isometrics.

**Q Are there any exercises I should avoid absolutely?**

A We wouldn't recommend the marathon, at least not right off the bat. And the blood pressure-raising strain associated with weight lifting is definitely out. Remember, moderation is the key.

One piece of equipment to avoid if you have moderate to high blood pressure is the inversion bar and shoes, or antigravity boots as they are sometimes called. What you do with this gear is simply hang upside-down. It's supposed to be good for the spine and the body's musculature, and some enthusiasts love doing sit-ups and other exercises while dangling from the bar like a bat. Inversion therapy is bad news, however, even for healthy, non-hypertensive people. After only three minutes of this 'suspended inanimation', even those with normal blood pressure have readings of 150/100.

## QUESTIONS AND ANSWERS

**Q  If I have high blood pressure, do I have to give up driving?**

A  Probably not. The research into this area hasn't shown any particular hazards either to drivers or to others. If you are hypertensive and find driving particularly stressful, however, you might be well advised to use some other form of transportation. You will certainly save aggro – you might even save some money.

**Q  And how about sex?**

A  Sexual intercourse has a great elevating effect, not the least of which has to do with blood pressure. Systolic blood pressure levels can more than double, diastolic rise by as much as 60 per cent, and heart rate increase to 120 per cent faster than usual. Some people have had coital blood pressures of 300/175 mm Hg, or 237/138 on average for men and 216/127 for women. The peak is reached at orgasm; less than 2 minutes later, blood pressure has receded to levels lower than those before sex. Higher levels are liable to occur when a person is having sex with a new partner.

This is not a thing we can give general advice on – every case is different, and people have different needs and priorities. Your doctor can best answer your questions about how safe having sex is for you.

**Q  I'm a smoker. Should I stop if I have high blood pressure?**

A  You should stop even if you haven't got high blood pressure, but especially if you have. There's enough evidence to point an accusing finger at smoking as one of the major risk factors in the development of high blood pressure, and as a real risk factor in accelerated **cardiovascular disease**.

Studies have shown that, while no one knows for certain exactly how tobacco smoke causes vascular disease, it's pretty clear that smoking causes the body to release more **catecholamines** into the system. Catecholamines are chemicals the body produces in response to stress. They make the heart beat faster and with greater force, and cause blood vessels to constrict, among other things. This increase in **cardiac output** raises the blood pressure. Smoking speeds up the release of the hormone **vasopressin**, and this too elevates blood pressure.

Researchers have shown that if a person inhales nicotine-containing smoke, the production of **prostacyclin** – a chemical that dilates, or expands, the openings of blood vessels – is reduced. By doing so, nicotine smoke is directly involved in higher blood pressure and, perhaps, more extensive coronary heart damage.

If that weren't enough, yet another study has demonstrated a connection between smoking and blockage of the kidney's artery (**renal artery stenosis**, to use the technical terminology). Scientists have known for many years that narrowing of the kidney arteries results in the production of a hormone which causes blood pressure to shoot up.

Finally, another recent study showed that nearly three-fourths of women who had been hospitalized for malignant hypertension were smokers and/or used oral contraceptives.

What this says, clearly, is that if you discover you have high blood pressure, giving up smoking has got to be one of the first steps you take. Giving it up before you develop the condition is better still. Best of all is never to start smoking to begin with. An ounce of prevention is worth a pound of hypertension.

Q **Wait a second – did you mention that oral contraceptives can cause high blood pressure?**

A Yes. Progestogen, an oestrogen in 'the pill', causes the body to produce more of a substance called angiotensin, which in turn elevates blood pressure. Oral contraceptives raise blood pressure in almost all women who take them, but more so in women with a family history of high blood pressure or those with a history of hypertension during pregnancy.

If there's any good to be said about all this, it's that 'pill'-produced high blood pressure is usually reversible – all you have to do is stop taking the oral contraceptive. A study in England found that women who had stopped using the pill for at least a month had blood pressures similar to those women who had never used the Pill.

If you plan to take the Pill, it's a good idea to have your blood pressure measured before you start. If it's already high, it may be wise to explore alternative methods of contraception. If your blood pressure is normal before using the Pill, doctors suggest checking your pressure regularly at home or at least every three to four months at the doctor's surgery for the first year of use. If everything's OK at that time, a twice-yearly checkup ought to do the trick. If your blood pressure is found to have risen, however, you will probably be advised to stop using the Pill.

**Q** **Well, now that I know that smoking and the Pill are probably bad for my blood pressure, what else do I have to look out for?**

**A** If you drink alcoholic beverages, you might want to reconsider the ways you wet your whistle.

**Q** **You mean you're going to take booze away from me, too?**

**A** No. You have to take it away from yourself. The evidence is fairly strong that those who tipple may topple.

When 4,783 men and women 20 years of age and older were studied by a team of scientists at the University of California at San Diego to see how drinking affected their blood pressure, the results (published in the journal *Hypertension*) indicated that as little as the equivalent of two doubles of spirits (four units) was all it took to produce a 'modest but consistent' increase in both systolic and diastolic pressure readings. The researchers noted that men 35 years of age or older downing this amount of booze were nearly twice as likely to have high blood pressure as non-drinkers. And the direct correlation was also clear: Blood pressure was especially high if those examined had had alcohol during the previous 24 hours.

According to a doctor working with the Stanford Heart Disease Prevention Program, by increasing alcohol consumption from one to three drinks per day in men 50 to 74 years old, systolic pressure would rise just as much as if the body weight of those men had increased from 12 to 14 stone. He also offered the theory that if you have at least one or two drinks a day, and if you also have high blood pressure and are over 50, you should try abstaining for a while – your blood pressure could go down, thus saving you unnecessary medication and possible side-effects.

Exactly how and why alcohol affects blood pressure isn't known – it just does. And that's important to know.

Q **How do my eating habits affect my blood pressure?**
A What you eat – and how much – has a lot to do with where your blood pressure level resides.

As a general rule, obesity and high blood pressure go hand in hand. Obesity may cause high blood pressure, which in turn may cause cardiovascular disease, but – as with nearly everything in the study of blood pressure – the mechanism is not clear. In fact, it may not be there at all. Obesity and high blood pressure could be totally independent problems, merely existing side by side in the same person. While many scientific studies show that the blood pressure of certain overweight people drops when those people lose some weight, other studies have indicated that the hypertensive obese person may not be in any greater danger of heart attack and heart-related deaths than a non-obese hypertensive – in fact, the obese person may be in less danger. Others say that weight loss without antihypertensive drug therapy at the same time may have no real and lasting effect on individuals with mild hypertension.

The authoritative *Scientific American Textbook of Medicine* states that in the control of blood pressure, weight-reduction is the most effective non-drug measure. It certainly pays to lose weight if you are too heavy, whether or not it shows up immediately on your blood pressure scorecard. Besides looking and feeling better, you will probably live longer, too. According to the Society of Actuaries, if you are 30 per cent above average weight, your risk of dying from coronary disease, compared with people of average weight, is 44 per cent higher for men and 34 per cent higher for women. Whether that has to do with blood pressure is irrelevant, really. It has to do with living, and that should be sufficient motivation.

**Q Are there any specific foods to stay away from?**
A Let's start by considering coffee.

For years debate has ensued on whether coffee, or caffeine intake, has an elevating effect on blood pressure. Early studies suggested that there was a close connection. One drew a clear connection between caffeine, high blood pressure and stress; it showed that a few cups of coffee can raise blood pressure, and when work-related stress or everyday pressures were factored in, the mixture wasn't good, especially for coffee-gulping, tense office workers. One researcher wrote in an issue of *Psychosomatic Medicine*: 'Blood pressure increases of the magnitude seen in the present study could potentially eliminate or reverse the therapeutic effects of a number of the antihypertensive drugs currently in use.' A more recent study – this one of more than 45,000 men by researchers at the Harvard University School of Public Health – exonerated coffee as a heart risk factor. The researchers reported in the *New England Journal of Medicine* that men who drank even as much as four cups of coffee a day had no higher risk of developing heart disease than those men who drank no coffee at all. The real problem with the early research was in the quality of the statistics. The figures may have been OK, but the interpretation of them probably was not. Tense people, prone to high blood pressure, are often just the kind of people who gulp down lots of coffee.

**Q How about meat?**

**A** The real problem with this question is that meat contains both protein and fats, and you can never completely separate them. In addition, some research which seemed to show a connection may have been flawed because the researchers looked at how vegetarians (who often have better blood pressure readings than omnivores) reacted to meat – never thinking that part of the observed blood pressure rise was the result of anxiety on the part of non-meat-eaters having to eat the stuff. However, at least one newer study took 'regular' eaters, put them on a vegetarian diet, watched as blood pressure dropped, put them back on their usual meals, and saw their blood pressure go back up again.

You needn't feel obliged to become a total vegetarian, but cutting down on meat is probably a good idea. The real point is that cutting down on meat means cutting down on fats, and it is the fats that matter.

**Q Is there more I should know about fats?**

**A** Certainly. When you need to use fats, use the polyunsaturated kind, like safflower, sunflower, corn, olive and canola oils (they may have a diuretic effect). Eat mackerel, rainbow trout, haddock and Atlantic salmon occasionally (they contain large amounts of eicosapentanoic acid – EPA – which is postulated to have a beneficial effect on blood pressure and cardiac health in general). Saturated fats – dairy and meat fats, the kind that are solid at room temperature – are very bad news. It's too simplistic to suggest that the fats get deposited directly in the linings of your arteries, but there is no doubt that a diet high in saturated fats is liable to increase your risk of cholesterol deposits in the arteries and the resulting high blood pressure.

**Q I gather fibre is a good thing. Which foods are high in dietary fibre?**

**A** So glad you asked:

## QUESTIONS AND ANSWERS

# FOODS HIGH IN DIETARY FIBRE

| Food | Portion Size | Grams of Fibre |
|---|---|---|
| 100% bran cereal | 1 cup | 19.9 |
| Baked beans | 1/2 cup | 8.3 |
| Apple | 1 medium | 7.9 |
| Broccoli, cooked stalk | 1 medium | 7.4 |
| Spinach, cooked | 1/2 cup | 5.7 |
| Almonds | 1/4 cup | 5.1 |
| Kidney beans | 1/2 cup | 4.5 |
| Cabbage, shredded, boiled | 1/2 cup | 4.3 |
| Shredded Wheat | 1 cup | 4.3 |
| Peas, cooked | 1/2 cup | 4.2 |
| Banana | 1 medium | 4.0 |
| Corn | 1/2 cup | 3.9 |
| Potato | 1 medium | 3.9 |
| Pear | 1 medium | 3.8 |
| Lentils | 1/2 cup | 3.7 |
| Lima beans, cooked | 1/2 cup | 3.5 |
| Sweet potato | 1 medium | 3.5 |
| Pinto beans | 1/2 cup | 3.1 |
| Peanuts, chopped | 1/4 cup | 2.9 |
| Brown rice, raw | 1/4 cup | 2.8 |
| Cornflakes | 1 cup | 2.8 |
| Oats, rolled | 1/2 cup | 2.8 |
| Orange | 1 medium | 2.6 |
| Raisins | 1/4 cup | 2.5 |

| | | |
|---|---|---|
| Brussels sprouts | 4 | 2.4 |
| Peanut butter | 2 tbs | 2.4 |
| Whole wheat bread | 1 slice | 2.4 |
| Apricots | 3 medium | 2.3 |
| Carrots, raw | 1 medium | 2.3 |
| Beets | ½ cup | 2.1 |
| Peaches | 1 medium | 2.1 |
| Kale, cooked | ½ cup | 2.0 |
| Courgettes, raw | ½ cup | 2.0 |

**Q And what about salt? That's supposed to be bad for me, isn't it?**

A Well, as we've been seeing, nothing's easy to say for sure when it comes to blood pressure. The subject of salt in the diet is another uncertainty that's grown into a full-blown controversy – one that's been brewing for nearly 80 years.

To start off with, the mineral sodium is necessary for human wellbeing. Sodium is a part of many foods and food additives. Salt is 40 per cent sodium, and salt is the vehicle by which most of us get our daily portion of sodium. The problem is this: Our daily portion is just too high. We only need 200 milligrams (mg) a day, but most of us are taking as much as 30 times that amount.

Most of us don't have any adverse reaction to sodium. However, it's likely that there is a large minority of people who are genetically programmed to react to sodium by having their blood pressure rise.

If we have learned anything in this book, it is that nobody knows for sure the mechanism for anything that has to do with blood pressure – and the sodium – high blood pressure connection is no exception. Some scientists believe that blood pressure goes up in the people in which it does go up because sodium increases water retention, and the result is greater arterial pressure. But that's just conjecture at the moment.

There's no real controversy about salt/sodium in some way causing high blood pressure in people genetically susceptible to sodium's effects. The argument has to do with the idea that by cutting back on sodium via low-salt diets, we can all avoid getting high blood pressure. There is no clear evidence that this is actually the case.

In other words, salt will more than likely raise your blood pressure if you already have high blood pressure (although this won't happen in all hypertensives), but it won't necessarily raise your blood pressure if you're **normotensive** (have blood pressure in the normal range).

Q So that settles it? Salt's not so bad after all?
A Unfortunately, the matter is far from settled. Some authorities insist that excessive sodium intake is a real cause for concern. Some suggest that the link between salt intake and raised blood pressure has been dangerously underestimated. It is clear, however, that although reducing one's salt intake may improve the effectiveness of drugs for hypertension, reduced salt intake, by itself, lowers the blood pressure in only 30–50 per cent of patients.

More worrying is the suggestion that low-sodium diets can actually increase some other cardiovascular risk factors. It can increase both insulin levels and the levels of low-density lipoproteins – the bodies that are known to carry cholesterol to the arteries. In addition, the important class of blood pressure-reducing drugs, the calcium channel blockers, are reported to be ineffective if the patient is also on a low-salt diet

A study conducted in the Netherlands involving newborn babies put half of the group of infants on a normal-sodium diet for the first six months of their lives, while the rest ate a low-sodium menu. Results: The normal-sodium babies developed higher blood pressure than the lower-sodium group, leading the doctors conducting the study to conclude that blood pressure is related to sodium intake and that 'moderation of sodium intake, starting very early in life, might perhaps contribute to prevention of high blood pressure and of rise of blood pressure with age.'

**Q** **So who's right and who's wrong?**
**A** Possibly everybody's a little right and perhaps everybody's a little wrong ... maybe.

**Q** **It's all so confusing – what's a person to do?**
**A** A concerned person will be careful, not overdo, and eat discriminatingly. The person with high blood pressure will go on a low-salt diet and see if that helps. It could help so much that further therapies, including antihypertensive drugs, will not be necessary, especially if yours is

a mild hypertension and you couple salt/sodium reduction with weight loss.

The person with normal blood pressure will control the urge to add salt to everything – just in case. Besides, food tastes better without extra salt. It tastes like itself. That's not to say you should abstain or put yourself through the boredom of a totally bland diet. A very low-salt diet is not only frustrating – eating tasty food is one of life's great pleasures – but it also ensures the urge to cheat, indulge, binge and, perhaps, pay the consequences ...

Q **Besides keeping the salt cellar off my table, what else can I do to restrict the sodium in my diet?**
A Here's what:

- Watch for the 'hidden' sodium in tinned, frozen or otherwise processed foods. Tinned vegetables often have salt added to them. Even tinned fruits may have salt in them.
- Don't go to all the trouble of keeping the cellar invisible while dining – then go and add salt to soups, stews, etc. while cooking. It does the same damage (that is, if it does damage). And make sure the same goes for when you eat out. All your willpower at the table can be for naught if the chef is going mad with the salt in the kitchen, or is using flour with a high sodium content, along with sodium-laden baking powder and baking soda. And if you're in a Chinese restaurant, be aware that the food is

often liberally spiced with monosodium glutamate (MSG), and this popular flavour-enhancer has a high sodium content. Furthermore, don't add soy sauce – Chinese or Japanese (tamari) – to the food; both have lots of sodium and 'hidden' MSG in them.

- Certain antacids are high in sodium, although in recent years new lines of antacids have been developed which are lower in sodium than their older cousins. Always check the label.
- Naturally occurring sodium can slip into your system unbeknownst to even the most scrupulous dietitians. One of the least expected is that found in milk (120 mg per cup). Celery, artichokes and spinach have moderate amounts of sodium too.
- Some drinking water may have a lot of natural sodium in it, but studies are inconclusive when it comes to whether this type raises your blood pressure significantly.
- Be sure you understand the language of low-salt. In one widely used standard, 'sodium-free' means less than 5 mg of sodium per serving; 'very low sodium' means 35 mg or less per serving; 'moderately low sodium' means 140 mg or less per serving; 'reduced sodium' means the usual level of sodium has been cut by at least 75 per cent; and 'unsalted', 'no salt added' or some equivalent phrase refers to food once processed with salt but now produced without it – although the food may contain other forms of sodium.
- Become expert at fixing your meals with spices

which will make you forget that there is even anything called sodium. For example:

- On eggs, try dill, oregano or chopped chives, individually or mixed together.
- For mashed potatoes, boil the potatoes with a clove of garlic, mash the potatoes, add chopped parsley, cayenne pepper, paprika, dill or curry powder.
- Season vegetables with nutmeg.
- Rub chicken with garlic, sprinkle with lemon juice and dust with paprika, sage and thyme.
- Rub red meats with fresh ginger and add rosemary or crushed black pepper.
- Dump out the salt from the salt cellars and fill them with oregano, basil, thyme, caraway seeds, sesame seeds or poppy seeds.
- Other spices to experiment with are allspice, chilli powder, curry, ground mustard, peppermint, tarragon, coriander, cardamom, cumin, cloves and celery seeds.

Q **Any other things good for me to eat for my high blood pressure?**

A Besides what's been discussed already, foods rich in the three minerals calcium, magnesium, and potassium — and high in their ratio to sodium — are generally conceded to be blood pressure-lowerers and heart-protectors.

Let's take calcium first. Results of one study point to the importance of calcium in the workings and the therapy of hypertension. Other research – and there is a good deal of it – has shown that hypertensives eat less calcium than normotensives; that when as many as 17 different nutrients were examined, it was only the calcium level that separated the high blood pressure sufferers from those with normal blood pressure; that a group of people without high blood pressure who added 1 gram (1,000 milligrams) of calcium to their daily diets had drops in their diastolic blood pressures; and that some scientists think that the way doctor-prescribed diuretics lower blood pressure is by increasing serum calcium levels. The evidence that calcium is an antihypertensive, when taken at daily levels of about 1,000 to 1,500 mg, is quite convincing.

The major report supporting the benefits of these three minerals – that of the American Joint National Committee on Detection, Evaluation and Treatment of High Blood Pressure – does not recommend that they should be taken in increased quantities, but simply that you should ensure that they are present in adequate amounts in your diet. Recommended daily amounts are:

| | |
|---|---|
| Potassium | 3000–3200 mg per day |
| Calcium | 800–1000 mg per day |
| Magnesium | 350–400 mg per day |

Here is a chart showing foods high in calcium which are also low in sodium:

# FOODS HIGH IN CALCIUM
## (AND LOW IN SODIUM)

| Food | Portion Size | Calcium (mg) | Sodium (mg) |
|---|---|---|---|
| Swiss cheese | 2 oz | 544 | 148 |
| Yoghurt (skim milk) | 1 cup | 452 | 174 |
| Yoghurt (low-fat) | 1 cup | 415 | 159 |
| Milk, skim | 1 cup | 302 | 126 |
| Milk, low-fat | 1 cup | 297 | 122 |
| Tofu | 4 oz | 145 | 8 |
| Blackstrap molasses | 1 tbs | 137 | 19 |
| Cabbages, cooked | ½ cup | 110 | 18 |
| Kale, cooked | ½ cup | 103 | 24 |
| Mustard greens | ½ cup | 97 | 13 |
| Watercress (chopped) | ½ cup | 95 | 33 |
| Almonds | ¼ cup | 83 | 1.5 |
| Salmon, fresh | 4 oz | 79 | 60 |
| Chick-peas, dried | ¼ cup | 75 | 13 |
| Broccoli | ½ cup | 68 | 8 |

**Q** And magnesium? Is that as effective as calcium?

**A** Yes. Study after study from all over the world shows that daily doses of magnesium, either through supplementation or in the diet, can keep blood pressure in its place.

The accompanying list offers most good food sources of magnesium. But, depending on your diet, you might feel that you need a supplement to be certain of getting at least the recommended daily allowance of 350–400 milligrams a day. If so, do keep in mind that magnesium works best when accompanied by about two times as much calcium. Also be alerted to the fact that so-called 'soft water' has fewer minerals in it than the 'hard' kind – and magnesium is among the missing. If your drinking water supply is 'soft' or softened, you might want supplementation all the more – because of the process involved, sodium levels are elevated in softened water, and studies show a greater amount of heart disease among inhabitants of communities where the water supplied is 'soft'. If you feel you have to take magnesium supplements – and very few people really need them – go easy on the dosage. Be careful to avoid excess.

## FOODS HIGH IN MAGNESIUM

| Food | Portion Size | Magnesium (mg) |
| --- | --- | --- |
| Soy flour, full fat | ½ cup | 180 |
| Tofu (soybean curd), raw | ½ cup | 127 |
| Almonds, not blanched | ¼ cup | 105 |
| Black-eyed beans, dried | ¼ cup | 98 |
| Soybeans, dry | ¼ cup | 98 |
| Wheat germ, toasted | ¼ cup | 91 |
| Cashews | ¼ cup | 89 |
| Brazil nuts, not blanched | ¼ cup | 79 |

| | | |
|---|---|---|
| Swiss chard, cooked | ½ cup | 75 |
| Rye flour | ½ cup | 74 |
| Whole wheat flour | ½ cup | 68 |
| Peanuts, dry-roasted | ¼ cup | 64 |
| Walnuts, black | ¼ cup | 63 |
| Peanut flour, defatted | ¼ cup | 56 |
| Oatmeal | 1 cup | 56 |
| Shredded wheat | 1 cup | 55 |
| Potato, baked | 1 medium | 55 |
| Blackstrap molasses | 1 tbs | 52 |
| Beet greens, cooked | ½ cup | 49 |
| Lima beans, baby, boiled | ¼ cup | 49 |
| Spinach, raw, chopped | 1 cup | 44 |
| Salmon, sockeye, tinned | 4 oz | 44 |
| Kidney beans, boiled | ½ cup | 40 |
| Avocado | ½ | 40 |
| Banana | 1 medium | 35 |
| Pecans, halved | ¼ cup | 35 |
| Milk, skimmed | 1 cup | 28 |
| Brown rice | ½ cup | 28 |
| Peanut butter | 1 tbs | 25 |
| Beef, round, lean | 3 oz | 24 |
| Chestnuts, roasted | ½ cup | 24 |
| Cabbages, cooked | 1 cup | 22 |

¹Source: *The Complete Book of Vitamins and Minerals for Health* (Rodale Press, 1988)

**Q  And potassium?**

**A**  Same story. Diets high in potassium seem to aid in the reduction of high blood pressure, particularly when the hypertension is also connected with sodium intake. Israeli scientists announced, after a good amount of research, that they felt that it was potassium which was the key antihypertensive agent in the vegetarian diet.

There are various theories as to how potassium works in keeping blood pressure down; nobody knows for sure, but it's felt that it acts as a diuretic, moving excess water from the blood vessel cell walls. In this way it is an antagonist of sodium, which works hard as a water-retainer. So lots of food scientists believe that foods high in potassium and low in sodium are very important for blood pressure control.

Here's a list of foods with a high potassium-to-sodium ratio, along with one that shows the opposite. Note that tinned and frozen foods aren't on the first list; that's because the canning and freezing processes change the potassium-to-sodium ratio in a negative way. For some eye-opening examples, see the list of processed foods.

# FOODS HIGH IN POTASSIUM (AND LOW IN SODIUM)

| Food | Portion Size | Potassium (mg) | Sodium (mg) |
|---|---|---|---|
| **Fresh vegetables** | | | |
| Asparagus | ½ cup | 165 | 1 |
| Avocado | ½ | 680 | 5 |
| Carrot, raw | 1 | 225 | 38 |
| Corn | ½ cup | 136 | trace |
| Lima beans, cooked | ½ cup | 581 | 1 |
| Potato | 1 medium | 782 | 6 |
| Spinach, cooked | ½ cup | 292 | 45 |
| Squash, winter | ½ cup | 473 | 1 |
| Tomato, raw | 1 medium | 444 | 5 |
| **Fresh fruits** | | | |
| Apple | 1 medium | 182 | 2 |
| Apricots, dried | ¼ cup | 318 | 9 |
| Banana | 1 medium | 440 | 1 |
| Cantaloupe | ¼ melon | 341 | 17 |
| Orange | 1 medium | 263 | 1 |
| Peach | 1 medium | 308 | 2 |
| Plums | 5 | 150 | 1 |
| Strawberries | ½ cup | 122 | trace |
| **Unprocessed meats** | | | |
| Chicken, light meat | 3 oz | 350 | 54 |
| Lamb, leg | 3 oz | 241 | 53 |

| | | | |
|---|---|---|---|
| Roast beef | 3 oz | 224 | 49 |
| Pork | 3 oz | 219 | 48 |

**Fish**

| | | | |
|---|---|---|---|
| Cod | 3 oz | 345 | 93 |
| Flounder | 3 oz | 498 | 201 |
| Haddock | 3 oz | 297 | 150 |
| Salmon | 3 oz | 378 | 99 |
| Tuna, drained solids | 3 oz | 225 | 38 |

# FOODS HIGH IN SODIUM (AND LOW IN POTASSIUM)

| Food | Portion Size | Potassium (mg) | Sodium (mg) |
|---|---|---|---|
| Salt | 1 tsp | trace | 2,132 |
| Soy sauce | 1 tsp | 22 | 1,123 |
| Bouillon cube | 1 | 4 | 960 |
| Cottage cheese (2 per cent fat) | ½ cup | 110 | 561 |
| **Hard cheeses** | | | |
| Parmesan | 2 oz | 53 | 1,056 |
| American | 2 oz | 93 | 812 |
| Brie | 2 oz | 87 | 356 |
| Muenster | 2 oz | 77 | 356 |
| Cheddar | 2 oz | 56 | 352 |
| Swiss | 2 oz | 64 | 148 |

## Snack foods

| | | | |
|---|---|---|---|
| Pretzels, thin, twisted | 10 | 10 | 1,008 |
| Potato crisps | 10 | 226 | 200 |
| Peanuts, roasted salted | ¼ cup | 243 | 151 |

## Processed meats

| | | | |
|---|---|---|---|
| Salami | 3 oz | 170 | 1,043 |
| Bologna | 3 oz | 133 | 981 |
| Frankfurter | 3 oz | 136 | 1,003 |

## Tinned soups

| | | | |
|---|---|---|---|
| Chicken noodle | 1 cup | 53 | 1,049 |
| Cream of mushroom (prepared with water) | 1 cup | 94 | 967 |
| Tomato | 1 cup | 247 | 816 |
| Vegetable beef | 1 cup | 162 | 896 |

## Tinned vegetables

| | | | |
|---|---|---|---|
| Beets | ½ cup | 142 | 200 |
| Corn | ½ cup | 80 | 195 |
| Lima beans | ½ cup | 188 | 200 |
| Peas | ½ cup | 82 | 200 |

The preparation of foods is crucial to the potassium-to-sodium ratio. For example, the potato is normally a good source of potassium – but when boiled, as much as 50 per cent of the potassium floats away ... and when boiled in salt water, nearly half the sodium in the water seeps into the potato.

Here's a look at various cooking preparations for a potato – and their results (*Na* is the symbol for sodium, *K* the symbol for potassium). As you can see, steaming is the hands-down winner.

| Cooking method | Na+ (mmol/l) | K+ (mmol/l) | K+/Na+ (ratio) |
|---|---|---|---|
| Raw | 1 | 104 | 104 |
| Boiled (peeled) in 1% salt | 90 | 64 | 0.7 |
| Boiled (peeled) unsalted | 1 | 79 | 79 |
| Boiled (unpeeled) in 1% salt | 30 | 84 | 2.8 |
| Boiled (unpeeled) unsalted | 1 | 94 | 94 |
| Steamed (peeled) unsalted | 1 | 100 | 100 |

## THE DIFFERENCE PROCESSING CAN MAKE

| | Portion Size | Potassium (mg) | Sodium (mg) |
|---|---|---|---|
| **Menu 1** | | | |
| Roast beef | 3 oz | 224 | 49 |
| Potato, baked | 1 medium | 782 | 3 |
| String beans, fresh | ½ cup | 95 | 2.5 |

| | | | |
|---|---|---|---|
| Whole wheat bread, firm crumb | 1 slice | 68 | 132 |
| Unsalted butter | 1 tbs | 4 | 1.4 |
| Peaches, fresh sliced | ½ cup | 172 | 1 |
| Milk, whole | 1 cup | 370 | 122 |
| Totals: | | 1,715 | 310.9 |

**Menu II**

| | | | |
|---|---|---|---|
| Corned beef | 3 oz | 51 | 802 |
| Potatoes, hash brown, frozen | 1 cup | 439 | 463 |
| String beans, tinned | ½ cup | 64 | 159.5 |
| White bread, soft crumb | 1 slice | 29 | 142 |
| Butter | 1 tbs | 3 | 140 |
| Peach pie | ⅛ pie | 176 | 316 |
| Milk, whole | 1 cup | 370 | 122 |
| Totals | | 1,132 | 2,144.5 |

**Q** **I have high blood pressure and my doctor's put me on medication. My blood pressure's gone down but I don't know how or why. What are these drugs and how do they work?**

**A** There are several classes of antihypertensive drugs and each works in a different way to alter body functions in order to control blood pressure. But we'll take them one at a time and explain the basics.

Before the basics, however, there is one thing about current blood pressure drug therapy that's important to remember: Many doctors practise a **stepped care** approach to the medication treatment of hypertension. That means that the doctor who recommends drugs for the control of high blood pressure – after exploring the use of other options such as weight loss, cutting out alcohol and smoking, and the various alternatives we've already mentioned – will usually start off a patient with the mildest of drugs at the smallest of doses, only gradually increasing the dosage of that drug to its maximum, and then introducing if necessary another, stronger drug at its mildest dose (alone or usually in combination with the drug used before it). The doctor will then gradually increase this second drug to its maximum, and may move on to another type of drug and increase it until the blood pressure is at a safe level and is stabilized. It's like a series of staircases, with each flight of stairs a different drug. Once you've climbed to the top of one, you start at the bottom of the next. With any luck, and in combination with other risk-reducing activities, you might need to go only a little way up that very first flight of stairs.

And another thing to remember: Step-down is the natural goal of a step-up approach – withdrawing the stronger drugs slowly as the blood pressure level stays firm.

Q **Which medication is the one to start with?**
A Ordinarily, and unless the blood pressure is dangerously high and immediate reduction is a matter of life and death, the first type of drug most often prescribed by doctors is a **diuretic**. Diuretics promote frequent

urination – it's no mystery, then, why many people refer to them as water pills – which increases the elimination of water and sodium from the body, and decreases the blood volume, among other things. The diuretics most often prescribed are members of the **thiazide** family – Aprinox, Dytide and Hydrenox are a few of the many popular brand names – except for so-called loop diuretics, which are used for high blood pressure cases related to kidney disease.

At a minimum, 40 to 50 per cent of people with high blood pressure who go on a drug regimen can control the disease with diuretics alone, and should begin to see results in six to eight weeks, or sooner.

Diuretics, *as do all other blood pressure medications*, have side-effects. The most frequent unwanted results of diuretic therapy are potassium deficiency, worsening of gout, and a rise in levels of cholesterol. The potassium problem may be overcome by taking supplements in doses recommended by your GP, by reducing sodium intake, or by using salt substitutes that contain potassium chloride. Orange juice or a banana or two a day probably aren't enough to prevent the deficiency, as is believed by many people. Gout flare-up is treated with yet another drug. And the cholesterol problem is fought by observing a low-fat diet.

Q  **What's the next series of drugs?**
A  In a typical programme of stepped care, if diuretics don't do the job, **adrenergic suppressants** or **inhibitors** are called into service. These include the drugs

propanolol (Inderal is the popular brand name version), nadalol (or Corgard) and metroprolol (Lopressor), all three of these being in the category known as beta blockers; clonidine (Catapres), methyldopa (Aldomet) and prazosin (Hypovase), and drugs containing **reserpine**.

Adrenergic suppressants differ from diuretics in one major regard: Whereas diuretics affect blood pressure through indirect means — by reducing sodium, water, and blood volume — adrenergic suppressants act directly on the heart, blood vessels and sympathetic nervous system. In general, they block the action of adrenaline — which, when pumped into the bloodstream in times of stress, causes elevations in heartbeat, cardiac output and blood pressure levels — and of the catecholamine noradrenaline.

There are many side-effects to look for in this group of drugs. Commonly occurring are depression, fatigue and impotence. Since there are so many side-effects specific to each one of these medications, a person who is prescribed any of them ought to ask the doctor or chemist for informational sheets on side-effects, dangers and contraindications. You can also ask your local librarian for a book on prescription drugs, or consult such a book in the reference section of the library.

Q Is there another 'step' up?
A Yes. The third level of drugs in a standard stepped care approach is that of the **peripheral vasodilators**, chief among them being hydralazine (popularly marketed

under the brand name Apresoline). These cause the peripheral blood vessels to widen to allow less restricted, less resistant blood flow. Again, if you find yourself being prescribed this type of medication, get a complete list of instructions, hazards and contraindications, and double-check with any information you can find in the library.

**Q** **Is that the last of the steps?**
**A** No. By the time you've reached this staircase, the climb has placed you in a group of only 5 per cent of people whose blood pressure has not responded well to treatment. There are even stronger drugs, and these will surely be prescribed, alone or in concert with other types.

**Q** **What you seem to be saying here is that drug therapy has been the turning point in the control of high blood pressure and the saving of lives. Is that right?**
**A** What we're saying is this: There's no question that the discovery and availability of many prescription antihypertensive medications are the reasons a lot of us are up and about today. They have played critical roles in the wellbeing of many sick people. But they should not be placed on a pedestal or given any special reverence. In fact, a marked decline in high blood pressure deaths has been going on since 1940 – and that's long before these drugs were even being dispensed. They are not *the* answer, just *an* answer, and maybe only the current answer ... tools to be used when the machinery calls for

it. And lately they're a tool a lot of doctors and scientists are thinking twice about before using.

**Q Really? Why – is there something wrong with them?**
**A** Well, beyond the very evident side-effects involved with the taking of many of these drugs – side-effects which may outweigh the benefits of the medication, or make life seem less worth living – there is some very serious debate going on about what to take and when, for how long, and if there are long-lasting disadvantages associated with antihypertensive drug use.

**Q For instance ...?**
**A** For instance the idea, long circulated among medical practitioners, that once you go on blood pressure drug therapy you've got to keep taking the pills for the rest of your life or pay mortal consequences.

More recently, some researchers have been reappraising this theory – especially in the light of the potential toxic effects of some of these drugs over the years.

Research has shown that nearly two-thirds of patients who are eased off their medication – at the same time that they institute some basic lifestyle changes – still have normal blood pressure after a year and a half. These are people with 'mild' hypertension, with diastolic readings of between 90 and 104. An interesting postscript to the study is that even those whose blood pressure can't be held down without returning to using medication are able to maintain normal pressure with dosages lower than before.

A study from the Hypertension Detection and Follow-up Program at the University of Mississippi School of Medicine showed pretty much the same results, and concluded that mild hypertensives whose blood pressure is being controlled by one drug and who are willing to modify their diet are prime candidates for a programme involving the elimination of that drug.

So, it seems, it's possible to be weaned off pressure-lowering medication with impressive results, if you're also willing to lose some weight, stop smoking, lower your sodium and alcohol intake and exercise more.

It would, needless to say, be unwise to do this on your own initiative, without first discussing it with your doctor.

Q **Very interesting. What else?**
A 'What else' is even more interesting.

The first 'what else' is a rethinking of using diuretics as the first flight in the stepped care approach. Many concerned doctors and scientists think that these diuretics are more toxic to the body's system in the long run, and create more (and, possibly, more life-threatening) adverse effects than any other antihypertensive medication; and, besides, the risk of potassium deficiency is more serious than it is often made out to be. These medical professionals are now thinking that a beta blocker might be better for a first, effective, and less toxic step.

But the big news is that a growing number of medical people (but still, unfortunately, within the minority) are coming round to the view that the key to therapy is not removing drugs once they've been started, but in not prescribing them in the first place – especially for people diagnosed as having mild hypertension (those with diastolic pressures between 90 and 104, a group which makes up about 75 per cent of people with high blood pressure).

These doctors and researchers suggest that no studies have made strong cases for the use of drugs in what is called 'uncomplicated' mild high blood pressure. What complicates matters are other cardiovascular risk factors muddying up the hypertension waters – things like smoking, diabetes, high cholesterol levels, family history, gender (males are more at risk), and race (black people are in greater danger than white people); these factors may add up to a need for some sort of drug therapy. But for most mild high blood pressure, there's no urgency to rush into pill-popping.

Your medical practitioner might not be up on his or her reading, and might not be following this latest move away from knee-jerk prescribing. It *is not* impolite, tactless, impertinent or out of place to bring up these matters. After all, *you* are the one taking – or not taking – the pills.

**Q** **What if your blood pressure doesn't improve after using the strongest of the drugs?**

**A** Sadly, some people's blood pressure just can't be controlled, and they die from the disease. Even more sadly, a number of these deaths could have been prevented because the failure is not in the drug but in the person taking it – or, rather, not taking it. In many cases, worsened conditions and fatalities are the result of people not taking their medication or not taking it in the proper manner.

If, however, a person is complying with the drug regimen and his or her blood pressure is still high, it is quite possible they are suffering from a case of overlooked secondary hypertension, and the doctor ought to redouble efforts to discover the underlying physical cause of the problem. Such cases deserve full investigation in hospital under the care of a consultant physician.

Q **Can high blood pressure be cured surgically?**
A When kidney troubles are at the root of the problem, surgery to unblock clogged renal arteries or transplants to give the body a healthy kidney often do the job, as do other procedures.

Q **Even though a low blood pressure reading is desirable, when is blood pressure too low? And what are the dangers of low blood pressure?**
A The medical term for **low blood pressure** is **hypotension**. According to at least one doctor, writing in the *New England Journal of Medicine*, 'Hypotension is not a disease; it is an ideal blood pressure level.' Furthermore, a cardiologist was quoted in the *British Medical Journal* as saying that 'the distribution of blood pressure in the population is such that a small percentage of people will have blood pressures well below the mean of the

general population.' In fact, the Framingham study – the Rolls Royce of cardiovascular risk factor reports – showed that as a general rule the lower the blood pressure, the longer you'll live (although the risk of cardiovascular disease is, oddly enough, somewhat higher for people with diastolic pressure around 70 mm Hg than for those with diastolic pressure around 90 mm Hg).

So long as you feel well with low blood pressure, it's OK. Hypotension is, however, a feature of various illnesses and conditions, including diabetes, **Addison's disease** and alcoholism. You can get sudden hypotension (leading to **syncope** – fainting – or even death) after exercise – which might be an indicator of undiscovered heart problems – or after spending time in a sauna. Hypotension is a principal characteristic of genuine shock.

Orthostatic (or postural) hypotension is a condition – sometimes leading to fainting – which occurs in many people when they sit or stand up suddenly after they've been lying down or sitting for a long time, especially after a spell in a sick bed. This type of hypotension, as well as the others, may have physical disorders as its root cause. However, it may also be **iatrogenic** in nature; that is, many people suffer hypotension because they've had hypertension and have begun taking medication – and the medication has brought their blood pressure down too low too fast ... occasionally even low enough to cause hypotensive stroke and death.

– often less invasive and with fewer side-effects than traditional medicine's – which has its adherents and apparent success stories.

It's an area of practice unfortunately engaged in by many who simply have no idea of the basic science of the subject, however. Regrettably, it also contains a few whose only real motive is to make money out of the gullible – but it is also an area of therapy which includes some dedicated people, some interesting ideas and some novel approaches. But be careful: Interesting ideas and novel approaches do not necessarily work. Beware of high prices, unusual and gimmicky machines allegedly designed to undo what's wrong with you, grandiose claims and other things that smack of the charlatan. So, *caveat emptor* – let the buyer beware – a piece of good old Latin advice to be applied when dealing with medical professionals as well.

Alternative treatment takes in a lot of territory – from acupuncture (practised by both doctors and medically unqualified people with some good results) to zone therapy, or reflexology, a type of treatment that uses massage of the hands and feet to influence the health and function of internal organs and systems.

A number of chiropractors feel that certain blockages of nerves responsible for normal circulation can be eliminated through manipulation techniques.

Practitioners of various massage methods – acupressure and shiatsu chief among them – report that some benefit is derived from their craft, if only that of rubbing away some tension and stress.

## QUESTIONS AND ANSWERS

**Q   When is a blood pressure reading considered low blood pressure?**

A   Again, it's a smudged line, but a person with low blood pressure is probably getting persistent readings of around 100/70 or less.

**Q   What can I do about my hypotension?**

A   As we said, if you feel all right, you don't have to do anything except congratulate yourself. If you don't feel all right, get yourself a checkup to see if the hypotension is indicative of a hidden condition. If you're on blood pressure medication, your doctor ought to look into scaling down the dosage. Ironically, you may have to do the very opposite of what people with high blood pressure do – you may be urged by your health practitioner to add more salt to your diet. If your problem is orthostatic or postural in nature, and blood doesn't reach your brain because it's pooling in your legs, you might want to start wearing tight, full-length, elastic support stockings.

**Q   Are there any alternative approaches to blood pressure treatment?**

A   Beyond the ones we've already talked about – diet, exercise, and behaviour modification – there are a variety of methods put forth by an assortment of alternative practitioners and alternative healers. While many of these practitioners can't produce the years of studies and double-blind experimental results that the medical professionals can, they none the less provide treatment

Homoeopathy, which in spite of its wholly illogical basis continues to be popular, provides harmless, limited-invasive treatment through administration of very small doses of homoeopathic drugs, salts and elements. Like other forms of unorthodox treatment, however, homoeopathy has no part to play in the management of potentially dangerous conditions such as hypertension.

Herbalists approach the treatment of high blood pressure by prescribing doses of traditionally used flowers, leaves and stems of a large number of plants, often prepared in the form of teas and other beverages. Unlike established drugs, herbal 'remedies' are not standardized. Some of them also contain potentially dangerous substances, and it's not too hard to get an overdose. Don't imagine that because a substance is 'natural' that it is necessarily safe. Deadly nightshade is natural.

Doctors of so-called natural healing techniques – naturopaths – may incorporate many of the aforementioned treatments in their practices, along with other nutritional advice. One of this discipline's longtime favourite remedies – eating lots of garlic – has been embraced (at least tentatively) by medical science as a high blood pressure curative and preventive agent.

The gentle, slightly cerebral exercise routines of yoga and t'ai chi help reduce blood pressure by taking the edge off, of stress. But don't try head-stands or shoulder stand poses – they will raise your blood pressure.

There are many practitioners – medical and alternative alike – who contend that many incidents of high blood pressure are the result of food allergies, and that finding and treating the allergy will end the hypertension. In fact, food allergy is far less common than the popular medical literature would suggest, and there is no reason to suppose that it has anything to do with high blood pressure.

It's definitely a crowded field, and a multifaceted one. Only experience, word-of-mouth recommendations or a good deal of background research can help you to select the method that's best for you ... if any is. It's a field that lacks consistency – finding two practitioners in the same discipline who will prescribe the same treatment for the very same condition is difficult; they promote their own tried-and-true 'sure things' – and it's a field that lacks the consistent reproducibility of results so important to making healing crafts credible. Still, people swear by them and sometimes seem to get well by them, and that's as much as can be said about a lot of medical doctors.

For people unhappy with the traditional medical approach, these alternatives are available for consideration. Many of them lend themselves to continued self-care, too.

Just remember that if you really have significantly raised blood pressure, you can't afford to take chances with methods of treatment with no proven basis. Medical science will never reject or neglect treatments which really do work and that are safe – whatever their nature.

The thing to remember is that at the end of the day

## QUESTIONS AND ANSWERS

you are in control of your own health and wellbeing. By looking after your weight, taking the right amount of exercise, eating the proper foods and generally keeping an eye on how you manage your lifestyle, you can in many cases help to keep your blood pressure under control.

# INFORMATION AND MUTUAL AID GROUPS

**British Heart Foundation**
14 Fitzhardinge Street
London W1H 4DH
0171–935 0185

**The Stroke Association**
CHSA House
Whitecross Street
London EC1V 8JJ
0171–490 7999

**American Heart Association**
7320 Greenville Avenue
Dallas, TX 75321
(214) 373–6300

**National Hypertension Association**
324 E. 30th Street
New York, NY 10016
(212) 889–3557

# GLOSSARY

**ACCELERATED HYPERTENSION**
   A particularly severe stage of high blood pressure. It is considered a medical emergency (blood pressure readings are quite high, especially the **diastolic**) that is often fatal in a very short time if left untreated. Related to kidney disease – either as cause or result – accelerated **hypertension** is a major cause of stroke

**ADDISON'S DISEASE**
   A chronic condition in which insufficient amounts of cortisone-like hormones are produced by the adrenal cortex. Incurable but controllable through replacement of deficient hormones, Addison's disease symptoms include a general feeling of weakness and fatigue, hypoglycaemia, gastrointestinal problems, and insufficient cardiac output. Mental and emotional problems also result

**ADRENERGIC SUPPRESSANT OR INHIBITOR**
   A type of antihypertensive drug that acts directly on the heart, blood vessels, and sympathetic nervous system

**AEROBIC EXERCISE**
   A type of vigorous physical activity designed to improve

the body's intake and utilization of oxygen. It is considered excellent exercise for improving cardiovascular health, and as a possible preventive of heart attacks and **high blood pressure**

## ATHEROSCLEROSIS

A common form of hardening of the arteries, this is a degenerative condition featuring accumulation of minerals and fatty deposits in the arteries, causing a rigidity and narrowing that affects the flow of blood through the body. Possible causes of atherosclerosis are high cholesterol levels in the blood, **high blood pressure** (which is, in turn, worsened by the continued thickening of the deposits and the ever-narrowing path for adequate blood flow), heredity, and stress, among others. Atherosclerosis is the number one killer of the Western world and is the principal cause of heart attacks and strokes

## BENIGN HYPERTENSION

A form of the disease that is not life-threatening; that is, it is not **accelerated** or **malignant**. It is still, however, a form that needs to be followed carefully and treated accordingly, because it can lead to worsening conditions and complications involving the eyes, the brain, the heart, and the kidneys

## BIOFEEDBACK

Information provided by various tools and methods that tells a person about any one or several body functions, the goal of which is to teach the person how to control those functions for better health. Biofeedback technology allows a person to hear or see his or her heartbeat

# GLOSSARY

or blood pressure or brain waves and, along with expert instruction, that person can learn to relax, become conscious of those physical states, and hopefully alter them

**BLOOD PRESSURE**

The force causing the blood's movement from the heart to and through the arterial **vascular system**, and the pressure of the blood expelled from the heart against the walls of the blood vessels it passes through

**BLOOD PRESSURE MACHINE**

The apparatus involved in taking a blood pressure measurement. See **Sphygmomanometer**

**BRACHIAL ARTERY**

The artery running down the length of the arm; under ordinary circumstances, it is used to help attain blood pressure measurements through use of the **blood pressure machine**

**CARDIAC OUTPUT**

A measurement of the volume of blood expelled by a ventricle of the heart. It is usually talked about in terms of volume of blood per minute

**CARDIOVASCULAR DISEASE**

The many and various diseases affecting the heart and blood vessels. See also **atherosclerosis, congestive heart failure, coronary artery disease, heart attack, stroke**

**CATECHOLAMINES**

Chemicals produced by the body that affect the way the body responds to stressful situations. The best known catecholamines are dopamine, adrenaline, and noradrenaline; by increasing cardiac output and constricting blood vessels, they work to increase the blood pressure

**CONGESTIVE HEART FAILURE**

A group of conditions involving a weak and failing heart and congestion, usually in the lungs. **High blood pressure** is a chief cause of congestive heart failure

**CORONARY ARTERY DISEASE**

Conditions and diseases involving the arteries that supply blood and oxygen to the heart

**DIASTOLIC**

That measurement of blood pressure when the heart is in its resting or relaxation phase, just before the next heartbeat. It is the 'lower number' in a blood pressure reading; that is, in a reading of 120/80, for example, the diastolic pressure is indicated by the 80

**DIURETIC**

A drug that promotes urination, thus speeding the elimination of water and sodium. This is an effective and much-prescribed method of blood pressure control

**ESSENTIAL HYPERTENSION**

A form of **hypertension** that makes up about 85 to 95 per cent of all high blood pressure cases. The cause is unknown – any one of many factors, including heredity and age, may be involved together or separately in affecting the way the body regulates pressure in the arteries – and it can be controlled but not cured

**HEART ATTACK**

A popular term for a destructive, often fatal event involving the heart. Medical names for this 'cardiac event' are *coronary thrombosis* and *myocardial infarction*.

# GLOSSARY

Both describe situations wherein a clot (occlusion) of some sort blocks up an artery, thus preventing blood to flow in its normal fashion. This, then, leads to the damage or death of heart muscle

## HIGH BLOOD PRESSURE
See **Hypertension**

## HYPERTENSION
A disease involving persistent high readings of blood pressure measurement. In general, when readings are taken over a period of time and show blood pressure greater than 140 mm Hg **systolic** and/or 90 mm Hg **diastolic** in people under age 40, that is high blood pressure, or hypertension; in people over 40, readings of 160 mm Hg systolic and/or 95 mm Hg diastolic or higher are considered indicative of hypertension

## HYPERTENSIVE HEART DISEASE
A disorder that occurs in people with **high blood pressure** when the heart, forced to work harder to pump blood through narrowed blood vessels, becomes enlarged. The pumping action of the heart is affected, and circulatory failure may follow

## HYPOTENSION
Low blood pressure. A person is usually considered hypotensive if he or she has continual blood pressure readings in which the **systolic** reading is less than 100 mm Hg

## IATROGENIC
Description of diseases or conditions that occur because of the actions of a doctor or another health care professional

# BLOOD PRESSURE

**ISOMETRIC EXERCISE**
A form of physical activity and bodybuilding that involves the application of bodily force against stable resistance

**LABILE HYPERTENSION**
High blood pressure that fluctuates and is not persistent. If untreated, labile **hypertension** can become persistent and health endangering. See *also* **Sustained hypertension**

**LEFT VENTRICLE**
A chamber of the heart on the lower left side. It pumps oxygenated blood into the circulatory system and body tissues

**LOW BLOOD PRESSURE**
See **Hypotension**

**MALIGNANT HYPERTENSION**
See **Accelerated hypertension**

**NORMOTENSIVE**
A term to describe a person whose blood pressure falls within normal, acceptable limits

**PERIPHERAL VASODILATORS**
A type of antihypertensive drug that works by widening the blood vessels to decrease resistance to blood flow

**PRIMARY HYPERTENSION**
See **Essential hypertension**

**PROSTACYCLIN**
A chemical in the body that acts as a vasodilator; that is, a blood vessel opener

# GLOSSARY

**PULSE PRESSURE**

A figure that indicates the difference between the **systolic** pressure and the **diastolic** pressure

**RENAL ARTERY STENOSIS**

A narrowing or obstruction of the kidney's artery

**RESERPINE**

A chemical used as a sedative and tranquillizer, and for the control of **high blood pressure**; derived from the dried root of any of the genus *Rauwolfia*

**RETINA**

A membrane at the back of the eye, it receives the images passed into the eye through the lens and sends them, via the optic nerve, to the brain. It is the only place in the human body where the small arteries (arterioles) can be looked at directly to see if any damage indicative of **hypertension** exists

**SECONDARY HYPERTENSION**

High blood pressure caused by some underlying disease or ailment. By eliminating the physical cause of secondary hypertension – for example, a kidney problem – it is often possible to bring the elevated blood pressure back to normal. In this way, it is unlike primary (**essential**) **hypertension**, which has no discernible cause

**SLEEP APNOEA**

An occasional, temporary stoppage of breathing while asleep, as a result of a failure of the autonomic nervous system to regulate the breathing. It leads to several conditions, among which is **high blood pressure**

**SPHYGMOMANOMETER**

The device most commonly used to measure **systolic**

and **diastolic** blood pressures. It allows notation and comparison of blood pressure levels by giving those levels values on a scale measured in millimetres (mm) of mercury (Hg)

## STEPPED CARE

A method of antihypertensive drug therapy that starts a **high blood pressure** sufferer on a low dose of a family of drugs and builds up dosage gradually in that and other families of drugs until control of pressure is achieved

## STROKE

A cerebral vascular accident wherein a ruptured or blocked blood vessel prevents blood from reaching important portions of the brain, leading to brain damage and subsequent debilitating conditions including paralysis and often death

## SUSTAINED HYPERTENSION

A description of high blood pressure that stays at the same high levels all the time and does not fluctuate to any important degree, as does **labile hypertension**

## SYNCOPE

Fainting, as a result of insufficient blood flow to the brain

## SYSTOLIC

That measurement of blood pressure when the left ventricle contracts and the blood's force against the vessel walls is at its greatest strength. It is the higher number in a blood pressure reading; that is, in a reading of 120/80, for example, the systolic pressure is indicated by the 120

# GLOSSARY

**THIAZIDE**
　A type of **diuretic** that works to reduce sodium, chloride, and water levels in the body through increased urination

**TINNITUS**
　A ringing, buzzing, roaring, or some other sort of noise in the ears that is long-term, distracting, dismaying, and often debilitating

**VASCULAR SYSTEM**
　The body's network of blood vessels

**VASOPRESSIN**
　A hormone secreted by the pituitary gland which, when released, causes the capillaries and arterioles to contract, resulting in an elevation of blood pressure

**VERTIGO**
　A sensation that makes a person feel as though either he or the world is spinning dizzily. It is often caused by **high blood pressure** or diseases of the inner ear, among other causes

# SELECTED BIBLIOGRAPHY

'Alcohol and hypertension', *Lancet* 24 June 1995: 1588

'Antihypertensive therapy: to stop or not to stop?' *Journal of the American Medical Association* March 27 1991: 1566–71

'Blood pressure measurement', *Lancet* 2 July 1994: 31

'Blood pressure and mortality', *Lancet* 1 April 1995: 825

'Caffeine and hypertension', *British Medical Journal* 16 November 1991: 1235

'Controlling hypertension with salt substitute', *British Medical Journal* 13 August 1994: 436

'Dietary salt and hypertension', *British Medical Journal* 5 April 1991: 811

'Does hypotension exist? *British Medical Journal* 11 Mar 1989: 660

'Epidemiology of hypertension', *Lancet* 9 July 1994: 101

'Exercise for hypertension', *Lancet* 15 May 1993: 1248

'Exercise training combined with antihypertensive drug therapy', *Journal of the American Medical Association* May 23–30 1990: 2766–71

'Failure of exercise to reduce blood pressure in patients

with mild hypertension', *Journal of the American Medical Association* October 16 1991: 2098–104.

'Genetics of hypertension', *Lancet* 9 May 1992: 1142

'Hyperlipidaemia, hypertension and coronary disease', *Lancet* 11 February 1995: 352

'Hypertension in the elderly', *Lancet* 13 August 1994: 447

'Hypertension octet (series of eight review papers on every aspect of the 'subject', *Lancet*, starting 2 July 1994: 31

'Hypertension in pregnancy', *British Journal of Hospital Medicine* 15 April 1992: 613

'Hypotension and chronic fatigue', *Lancet* 11 March 1995: 623

'Low blood pressure depression', *British Medical Journal* 12 February 1994: 446

'Low blood pressure – a disease?', *British Medical Journal* 18–25 August 1990: 362

'Management of hypertension in the elderly', *British Medical Journal* 26 September 1992: 750

'Management of hypertensive crises', *Journal of the American Medical Association* August 14 1991: 829–35.

'National education programs working group report on the management of patients with hypertension and high blood cholesterol', *Annals of Internal Medicine* February 1 1991: 224–36.

'Psychiatric symptoms and low blood pressure *British Medical Journal* 11 January 1992: 64

'Relaxation treatment for hypertension', *British Medical Journal* 26 May 1990: 1368

'Renal artery stenosis and hypertension', *Lancet* 23 July 1994: 237

'Renin and hypertension', *British Medical Journal* 27 April 1991: 981

'Salt and blood pressure', *British Medical Journal* 30 July 1988: 307

'Salt dominance in manufactured food', *Lancet* 21 February 87: 426

'Sex and hypertension', *British Journal of Sexual Medicine* February 1990: 58

'Smoking and blood pressure', *British Medical Journal* 12 January 1991: 89

'Steroids and hypertension', *Lancet* 23 July 1994: 240

'Stress and blood pressure', *British Medical Journal* 25 March 1995: 771

'Treating hypertension after stroke', *British Medical Journal* 11 June 1994: 1523

'Treating hypertension in the elderly', *British Medical Journal* 10 October 1992: 845

# INDEX

acetylcholine 8
acupressure 52
acupuncture 52
Addison's disease 50
aerobic exercise 16
age, diastolic pressure
    and 13
alcohol 20
alcoholism 50
Aldomet 44
alternative treatments 51
  caveats about 54
  warnings about 52
angiotensin 19
antihypertensive drugs 41
Apresoline 45
Aprinox 43
arm cuff 4
avoiding drugs 48

behaviour therapy 15
beta blockers 44
  depression and 44
  fatigue and 44
  impotence and 44
  side effects of 44
blood pressure
  ageing and 12
  alcohol and 20
  atherosclerosis and 12
  chronic anxiety and 13
  diastolic 2
  foods and 22
  hardening of arteries
    and 12
  how measured 3
  low 49
  measurement,
    accuracy of 5
  nervousness and 13

## BLOOD PRESSURE

  normal 3
  obesity and 21
  overeating and 21
  pulse 2
  salt and 26
  sexual intercourse and 17
  stress and 14
  surgical treatment of 49
  symptoms of 9
  systolic 1
  two levels 1
  uncontrollable 48
  what is high? 6
  what it is 1
blood pressure machine 4
blood pressure measurement
  at home 6
  cuff width 5
  digital devices 6
  reasons for inaccuracy 5
  repeated 6
  single readings inadequate 7
blurred vision 9

calcium 31
Catapress 44
catecholamines 18
chiropraxis 52
chronic anxiety 13
  blood pressure and 13
clonidine 44
coffee 22
contraceptive pill 19
Corgard 44
cuff width, blood pressure measurement 5

debate about drugs 46
diabetes 50
diastolic pressure 2
  age and 13
  significance of 3
dietary fats 24
dietary fibre 24
disadvantages of drugs 46
diuretic drugs
  potassium loss 43
  side effects 43
driving 17
drug treatment
  compliance with 49
  diuretics 42
  how to start 42

# INDEX

overdone 51
stepped approach 41
drugs
   adrenergic inhibitors 43
   avoiding 48
   beta blockers 44
   debate about 46
   disadvantages of 46
   diuretics 47
   how long to be taken? 46
   for hypertension 41
   limitations of 45
   low blood pressure and 50
   peripheral vasodilators 44
   substitutes for 46
   weaning off 47
Dytide 43

elastic support stockings 51
exercise 15

faintness on standing 50
fatigue 9
fats, dietary 24
food allergy 54
food seasoning without sodium 31
foods
   blood pressure and 22
   high calcium (table) 33
   high magnesium (table) 34
   high potassium (table) 37
   high sodium (table) 38
   preparation of 39
foods high in fibre (table) 25
Framingham study 50
frequency of hypertension 8

garlic 53
gout 43

headaches 9
head-standing 53
   danger of 53
heart enlargement 10
herbalism 53
   dangers of 53
heredity 10
high blood pressure
   acetylcholine and 8
   blurred vision and 9

- complications of 9
- consequences of 8
- ethnic incidence 11
- eye examination for 12
- fatigue and 9
- frequency of 8
- headaches and 9
- natriuretic hormone and 8
- nose bleeds and 9
- palpitations and 9
- seasons and 12
- sex ratio 11
- silent killer 8
- sleep apnoea and 8
- strokes and 9
- symptoms of 8
- tinnitus and 9
- weather and 12

homoeopathy 53
- danger of 53

hydralazine 44
Hydrenox 43
hypertension
- acetylcholine and 8
- benign 11
- blurred vision and 9
- causes of 7
- complications of 9
- consequences of 8
- drugs for 41
- ethnic incidence 11
- fatigue and 9
- frequency of 8
- headaches and 9
- labile 7
- natriuretic hormone and 8
- never really benign 11
- nose bleeds and 9
- palpitations and 9
- secondary 10
- sex ratio 11
- sleep apnoea and 8
- stress and 7
- strokes and 9
- sustained 7
- symptoms of 8
- tinnitus and 9

hypotension 50
Hypovase 44

Inderal 44
inversion bar 16
isometric exercise 16

kidney disease, hypertension and 10

# INDEX

labile hypertension 7
lifestyle management 55
limitations of drugs 45
Lopresor 44
low blood pressure 49
    how defined 51
    management of 51
low-density lipoproteins 28

magnesium 31, 33
massage 52
meat eating 23
methyldopa 44
metoprolol 44
minerals, recommended daily allowance of 32
monosodium glutamate 30
multifactorial aetiology 7

nadolol 44
natriuretic hormone 8
naturopathy 53
nervousness, blood pressure and 13
normal blood pressure 3
nose bleeds 9

obesity 21
oral contraceptives 19
orthostatic hypotension 50
overeating, blood pressure and 21

palpitations 9
potassium 31, 36
prazocin 44
progestogen 19
propranolol 44
prostacyclin 18
pulse pressure 2

reflexology 52
reserpine 44
retinal arteries 12
retinal examination 12

salt 26
    blood pressure and 26
salt in cooking 29
saturated fats 24
sexual activity 17
sexual intercourse, blood pressure and 17
shiatsu 52
shock 50
silent killer 8

sleep apnoea 8
smoking 17
Society of Actuaries 22
sodium 26
   in milk 30
   in vegetables 30
soy sauce 30
sphygmomanometer 3
   checking 6
   how used 4
stethoscope
   what is heard 4
   why used 4
stress 14
   blood pressure and 14
strokes 9
substitutes for drugs 46
surgical treatment of blood pressure 49
systolic pressure 1
  significance of 3

t'ai chi 53
taking control 55
thiazide drugs 43
tinnitus 9
transcendental meditation 15

undetected high blood pressure 10

vegetarian diet 23
ventricle 1

weaning off drugs 47
weight lifting 16
weight reduction 22

yoga 53

zone therapy 52

*Of further interest...*

# HEART DISEASE: QUESTIONS YOU HAVE ... ANSWERS YOU NEED

## KARLA MORALES

Heart disease is the leading cause of death in the Western world. In the light of this sobering statistic, it is essential to know as much as possible about your heart.

This vital guide cuts through the medical jargon and gives clear answers to hundreds of commonly asked questions:

- What causes heart disease?
- What happens during a bypass operation?
- Can heart disease be prevented?
- How dangerous is high blood pressure?
- What is a heart attack?

All the facts you need to know about heart health.

*The New Self Help Series*

# HIGH BLOOD PRESSURE

*Non-Drug Ways to Control Hypertension*

**LEON CHAITOW**

Explains the background and causes of high blood pressure (hypertension) and describes ways of tackling it through the use of self-help methods.

Simple alterations in diet, exercise and behaviour can quite often bring about dramatic change and lead towards the restoration of healthy function.

*Thorsons Health Series*

# HIGH BLOOD PRESSURE

*How to Lower Your Blood Pressure in Four Easy Stages*

**DR CAROLINE SHREEVE**

The number of people suffering from high blood pressure and heart attacks is on the increase – but there are preventive measures that can be taken. Here is a programme of drug-free ways to combat high blood pressure, which includes advice on what to eat, beneficial nutrition supplements and simple relaxation routines.

Dr Caroline Shreeve explains:

- the nature of your circulatory system
- factors responsible for regulating blood pressure
- the dangers accompanying high blood pressure
- why anti-hypertensive drugs are not the only answer.

She also gives guidance on the best forms of alternative or complementary therapy for reducing blood pressure and maintaining it within normal limits.

# HEART HEALTH FOR WOMEN

**FELICITY SMART AND DR DIANA HOLDRIGHT**

Coronary heart disease is a leading cause of disability and death among women, yet this has only recently been recognised. Previously, it was seen as being mainly a male problem, since it strikes many men at a younger age.

Although women become increasingly vulnerable after the menopause, risk factors earlier in their lives influence its development, and there is concern that many more younger women will be affected. It is therefore essential that every woman should be well-informed about heart disease.

This comprehensive book is the first for women which clearly explains its causes, symptoms, investigation and treatment. Most importantly, vital advice is given on prevention through healthy living, which also improves the outlook for those already affected.

A collaboration between two women with a keen interest in the subject – a cardiologist and a medical writer – this book will encourage all women to protect themselves and ensure that they receive expert help if necessary. Heart Health for Women is for those who care about having a healthier heart for life.

# RECIPES FOR HEALTH: HIGH BLOOD PRESSURE

**MAGGIE PANNELL**

Diet is becoming more and more popular as an effective way of treating, preventing and controlling the development of high blood pressure – hypertension – one of the most common and most serious of all health conditions.

Doctors recommend adopting a diet which is:

- low in salt
- calorie-controlled for weight reduction.

In this book, Maggie Pannell, an expert on food and nutrition, follows these dietary guidelines and presents delicious ways to reduce blood pressure and eat healthily. She explains the causes and dangers of the condition, suggests which foods to avoid and recommends eating less fat, less sugar and more fibre.

The recipes include exciting ideas for breakfasts, soups and starters, light meals, salads, main meals and desserts as well as a mouth-watering selection of menus for special occasions.

This book can really help to reduce your blood pressure safely – in the most enjoyable way!

# THE COMPLETE BOOK OF MEN'S HEALTH

## DR SARAH BREWER

Did you know?

- *80% of men will need treatment for prostate problems.*
- *The male sperm count has halved over the last 50 years.*
- *Your diet may be helping you go bald.*
- *Coronary heart disease is the biggest male killer.*

Men's health has been ignored for far too long. This is the first major book to deal with the subject in a comprehensive fashion, and includes important information on over 300 conditions from acne to erections, from irritable bowel syndrome to herpes.

This essential reference book for all men reveals crucial facts about your health, including:

- how to improve your sperm count
- how to decrease your risk of cancer
- how to decrease your risk of heart disease
- how to examine your testicles
- how to obtain enough exercise
- how changing your diet can protect against male diseases.

| | | | |
|---|---|---|---|
| **HEART DISEASE** | 0 7225 3312 8 | £3.99 | ☐ |
| **HIGH BLOOD PRESSURE: NEW SELF HELP** | 0 7225 1221 X | £2.99 | ☐ |
| **HIGH BLOOD PRESSURE:** | | | |
| **THORSONS HEALTH SERIES** | 0 7225 3041 2 | £5.99 | ☐ |
| **HEART HEALTH FOR WOMEN** | 0 7225 2992 9 | £6.99 | ☐ |
| **HIGH BLOOD PRESSURE:** | | | |
| **RECIPES FOR HEALTH** | 0 7225 3144 3 | £5.99 | ☐ |
| **COMPLETE BOOK OF MEN'S HEALTH** | 0 7225 3019 6 | £9.99 | ☐ |

All these books are available from your local bookseller or can be ordered direct from the publishers.

To order direct just tick the titles you want and fill in the form below:

Name: _____

Address: _____

_____

_____ Postcode: _____

Send to Thorsons Mail Order, Dept 3, HarperCollins*Publishers*, Westerhill Road, Bishopbriggs, Glasgow G64 2QT.

Please enclose a cheque or postal order or your authority to debit your Visa/Access account –

Credit card no: _____

Expiry date: _____

Signature: _____

– up to the value of the cover price plus:

**UK & BFPO:** Add £1.00 for the first book and 25p for each additional book ordered.

**Overseas orders including Eire:** Please add £2.95 service charge. Books will be sent by surface mail but quotes for airmail dispatches will be given on request.

**24-HOUR TELEPHONE ORDERING SERVICE FOR ACCESS/VISA CARD-HOLDERS — TEL: 0141 772 2281.**